The Vibrant Plant-Based Diet Cookbook

Enjoy your Meals with these Special Recipes

Luke Gorman

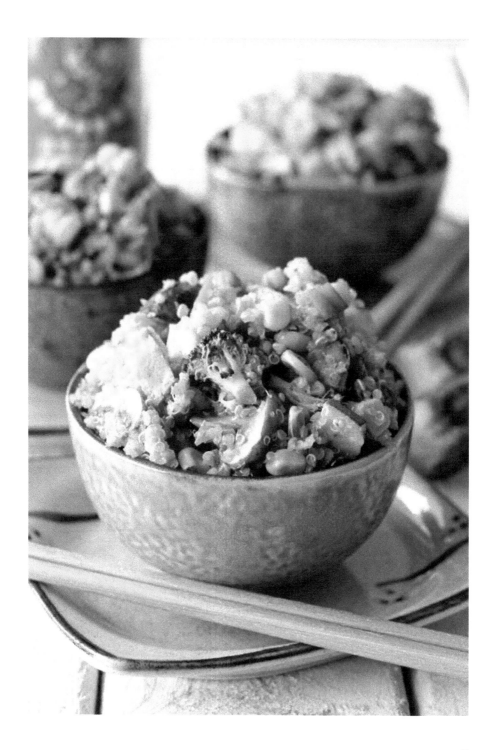

TABLE OF CONTENTS

Introduction

A plant-based eating routine backing and upgrades the entirety of this. For what reason should most of what we eat originate from the beginning?

Eating more plants is the first nourishing convention known to man to counteract and even turn around the ceaseless diseases that assault our general public.

Plants and vegetables are brimming with large scale and micronutrients that give our bodies all that we require for a sound and productive life. By eating, at any rate, two suppers stuffed with veggies consistently, and nibbling on foods grown from the ground in the middle of, the nature of your wellbeing and at last your life will improve.

The most widely recognized wellbeing worries that individuals have can be reduced by this one straightforward advance.

Things like weight, inadequate rest, awful skin, quickened maturing, irritation, physical torment, and absence of vitality would all be able to be decidedly influenced by expanding the admission of plants and characteristic nourishments.

If you're reading this book, then you're probably on a journey to get healthy because you know good health and nutrition go hand in hand.

Maybe you're looking at the plant-based diet as a solution to those love handles.

Whatever the case may be, the standard American diet millions of people eat daily is not the best way to fuel your body.

If you ask me, any other diet will already be a significant improvement. Since what you eat fuels your body, you can imagine that eating junk will make you feel just that—like junk.

I've followed the standard American diet for several years: my plate was loaded with high-fat and carbohydrate-rich foods. I know this doesn't sound like a horrible way to eat, but keep in mind that most Americans don't focus on eating healthy fats and complex carbs—we live on processed foods.

The consequences of eating foods filled with trans fats, preservatives, and mountains of sugar are fatigue, reduced mental focus, mood swings, and weight gain. To top it off, there's the issue of opening yourself up to certain diseases—some life-threatening—when you neglect paying attention to what you eat .

Mushroom and Quinoa Burger

Preparation time: 15 minutes

Cooking time: 40 minutes

Servings: 5

Ingredients:

For the Burgers:

- 1 cup cooked quinoa
- 4 medium caps of Portobello mushroom, gills removed, chopped
- 1/4 cup chopped red onion
- ½ teaspoon minced garlic
- 3 green onions, chopped
- 1/2 cup cornstarch
- 1/2 cup walnuts
- 2 teaspoons rice wine vinegar
- 2 tablespoons olive oil
- 5 whole-grain burger buns

For Toppings:

- Sprouts as needed

- Lettuce as needed
- Sliced tomatoes as needed
- Vegan mayonnaise as needed

Directions:

1. Prepare the burgers and for this, place mushrooms in a baking dish, add garlic and nuts, drizzle with 1 tablespoon oil, season with ¾ teaspoon salt and ¼ teaspoon black pepper, and then bake for 20 minutes until tender.
2. Then transfer the mushroom mixture in a food processor, add remaining ingredients for a burger, except for buns, stir until well mixed and then shape the mixture into five patties.
3. Fry the patties in batches for 5 minutes until browned and then bake for 10 minutes at 375 degrees F until thoroughly cooked.
4. Sandwich patties in burger buns, top with mayonnaise, sprouts, lettuce and tomatoes, and then serve.

Summer Minestrone

Preparation time: 5 minutes

Cooking time: 15 minutes

Servings: 4

Ingredients:

- 1 medium yellow squash, cut into 1/2-inch pieces
- 1/2 cup frozen peas
- 1 small carrot, peeled, sliced
- 1 small zucchini, cut into 1/2-inch pieces
- 8 ounces red potatoes, peeled, cut into 1/2-inch pieces
- 1 large onion, peeled, chopped
- 1 tablespoon olive oil
- 1 teaspoon minced garlic
- 1/3 teaspoon ground black pepper
- 2/3 teaspoon salt
- 1 cup chopped basil
- 4 cups vegetable broth
- 1/4 cup grated vegan parmesan cheese

Directions:

1. Take a large saucepan, place it over medium heat, add oil and when hot, add onion, stir in black pepper and salt and cook for 8 minutes.
2. Then stir in garlic, cook for 1 minute, stir in potatoes, pour in broth and simmer for 5 minutes.
3. Add carrot, squash, and zucchini, continue simmer for 3 minutes, and then add peas, simmer for another 3 minutes.
4. Stir in basil and cheese and then serve with bread

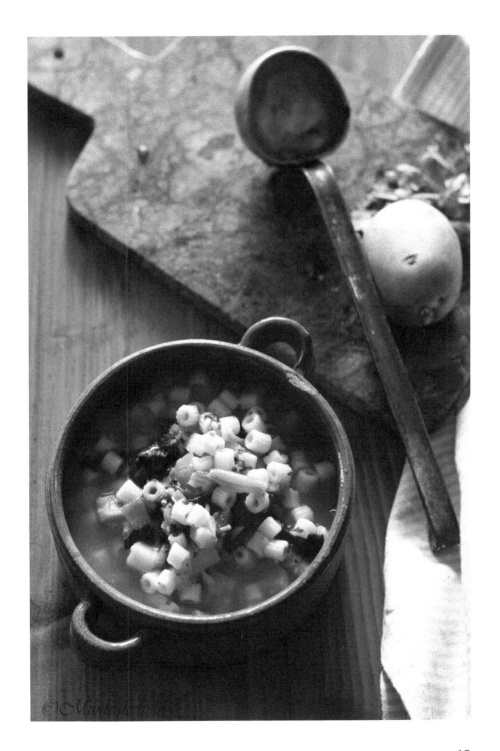

13

Veggie Kabobs

Preparation time: 10 minutes

Cooking time: 10 minutes

Servings: 10

Ingredients:

- 8 ounces button mushrooms, halved
- 2 pounds summer squash, peeled, 1-inch cubed
- 12 ounces small broccoli florets
- 2 cups grape tomatoes
- 1 teaspoon salt
- 1/2 teaspoon smoked paprika
- 1 teaspoon ground cumin
- 6 tablespoons olive oil
- 1/2 teaspoon ground coriander
- 1 lime, juiced

Directions:

1. Toss broccoli florets with 1 tablespoon oil, toss tomatoes and squash pieces with 2 tablespoons oil, then toss

mushrooms with 1 tablespoon oil and thread these vegetables onto skewers.

2. Grill mushrooms and broccoli for 7 to 10 minutes, squash and tomatoes and 8 minutes, and when done, transfer the skewers to a plate and drizzle with lime juice and remaining oil.

3. Prepared the spice mix and for this, stir together salt, paprika, cumin, and coriander, sprinkle half of the mixture over grilled veggies, cover them with foil for 5 minutes, and then sprinkle with the remaining spice mix. Serve straight away.

Linguine with Wild Mushrooms

Preparation time: 5 minutes

Cooking time: 3 minutes

Servings: 4

Ingredients:

- 12 ounces mixed mushrooms, sliced
- 2 green onions, sliced
- 1 ½ teaspoon minced garlic
- 1 pound whole-grain linguine pasta, cooked
- 1/4 cup nutritional yeast
- ½ teaspoon salt
- ¾ teaspoon ground black pepper
- 6 tablespoons olive oil
- ¾ cup vegetable stock, hot

Directions:

1. Take a skillet pan, place it over medium-high heat, add garlic and mushroom and cook for 5 minutes until tender.

2. Transfer the vegetables to a pot, add pasta and remaining ingredients, except for green onions, toss until combined and cook for 3 minutes until hot.
3. Garnish with green onions and serve.

Pilaf with Garbanzos and Dried Apricots

Preparation time: 10 minutes

Cooking time: 15 minutes

Servings: 4

Ingredients:

- 1 cup bulgur
- 6 ounces cooked chickpeas
- 1/2 cup Dried apricot
- 1 small white onion, peeled, diced
- ½ teaspoon minced garlic
- 2 teaspoons curry powder
- 1/2 teaspoon salt
- 1 tablespoon olive oil
- 1/4 cup fresh parsley leaves
- 2 cups vegetable broth
- 3/4 cup water

Directions:

1. Take a saucepan, place it over high heat, pour in water and 1 ½ cup broth, and bring it to a boil.
2. Then stir in bulgur, switch heat to medium-low level and simmer for 15 minutes until most of the liquid has absorbed.
3. Meanwhile, take a skillet pan, place it over medium heat, add oil and when hot, add onion, cook for 10 minutes, then stir in garlic and curry powder and cook for another minute.
4. Then add apricots, beans, and salt, pour in remaining broth and bring the mixture to boiling.
5. Remove pan from heat, fluff the bulgur with a fork, add to the onion-apricot mixture and stir until mixed.
6. Garnish with parsley and serve.

Brussels Sprouts

Preparation time: 10 minutes

Cooking time: 25 minutes

Servings: 1

Ingredients:

- 2 pounds Brussels sprouts, halved
- 1 teaspoon minced garlic
- ¾ teaspoon ground black pepper
- 1 tablespoon cornstarch
- 1 ½ teaspoon salt
- 1 tablespoon brown sugar
- 1/8 teaspoon red pepper flakes
- 1 tablespoon sesame oil
- 2 tablespoons olive oil
- 2 teaspoons apple cider vinegar
- 1/2 cup soy sauce
- 1 tablespoon hoisin sauce
- 2 teaspoons garlic chili sauce
- 1/2 cup water
- Sesame seeds as needed for garnish

- Green onions as needed for garnish
- Chopped roasted peanuts as needed for garnish

Directions:

1. Place sprouts on a baking sheet, drizzle with oil, season with salt and black pepper, and then bake for 20 minutes at 425 degrees F until crispy and tender.
2. Meanwhile, take a skillet pan, place it over medium heat, add oil and when hot, add garlic and cook for 1 minute until fragrant.
3. Then stir in cornstarch and remaining ingredients, except for garnishing ingredients and simmer for 3 minutes, set aside until required.
4. When Brussel sprouts have roasted, add them to the sauce, toss until mixed and broil for 5 minutes until glazed.
5. When done, garnish with nuts, sesame seeds, and green onions and then serve.

Stuffed Sweet Potato

Preparation time: 10 minutes

Cooking time: 45 minutes

Servings: 4

Ingredients:

- pounds sweet potatoes
- 1/3 cup corn kernels
- 1 cup chopped kale
- 1/4 cup diced green onion
- 3/4 cup diced tomato
- ½ teaspoon minced garlic
- 1/2 teaspoon sea salt
- 1/2 teaspoon chipotle flakes
- 1/2 teaspoon Dijon mustard
- 1/2 teaspoon smoked paprika
- 1/2 teaspoon liquid smoke
- 1/4 teaspoon ground turmeric
- 1/2 tablespoon lemon juice
- 3 tablespoons nutritional yeast
- 1/3 cup cashews, soaked, drained

- 1 1/2 cup pasta, cooked
- 1 cup baked pumpkin puree
- 1/2 cup vegetable broth

Directions:

1. Wrap each potato in a foil and then bake for 45 minutes at 375 degrees F until tender.
2. Meanwhile, prepare the cheese sauce and for this, place pumpkin and cashews in a food processor, add garlic, yeast, salt, paprika, chipotle flakes, liquid smoke, turmeric, mustard, and lemon juice, pour in broth and puree until smooth.
3. Take a pot, place it over medium-low heat, add prepared sauce, then add remaining ingredients, toss until coated, and cook for 5 minutes until kale has wilted.
4. Season the mixture with salt and black pepper, then switch heat to the low level and cook until sweet potatoes have roasted.
5. When sweet potatoes are roasted, let them stand for 10 minutes, then unwrap them, split them by slicing down the center and spoon prepared sauce generously in the center.
6. Serve straight away.

Tofu Tikka Masala

Preparation time: 10 minutes

 Cooking time: 4 hours and 10 minutes

Servings: 4

Ingredients:

- 16 ounces tofu, extra-firm, drained,
- ½ inch cubed
- 1 ½ teaspoon minced garlic
- 2 medium carrots, peeled sliced
- 1 medium white onion, peeled, diced
- 1 1/2 cups diced potatoes
- 1 medium red bell pepper, cored, cut into chunks
- ¾ cup frozen peas
- 2 cups cauliflower florets
- ½ tablespoon grated ginger
- ¼ teaspoon ground black pepper
- ½ teaspoon salt
- ½ teaspoon ground turmeric
- 1 ½ teaspoons cumin
- ¼ teaspoon cayenne pepper

- 1 tablespoon garam masala
- 1 teaspoon coriander
- ¼ teaspoon paprika
- ½ tablespoon maple syrup
- 15 ounces tomato sauce
- 15 ounces of coconut milk
- 2 tablespoons chopped cilantro

Directions:

1. Take a slow cooker, place all the ingredients in it, except for cilantro and peas, and stir until combined.
2. Switch on the slow cooker, shut with lid, and cook for 4 hours at a high heat setting.
3. When done, stir in peas, cook for 10 minutes, uncovering the cooker, and, when done, serve with cooked brown rice.

Buffalo Cauliflower Tacos

Preparation time: 10 minutes

Cooking time: 20 minutes

Servings: 4

Ingredients:

For the Cauliflower:

- 1/2 head cauliflower, cut into florets
- 1 teaspoon garlic powder
- ¼ teaspoon ground black pepper
- 1 teaspoon red chili powder
- 4 teaspoons olive oil
- 3/4 cup buffalo sauce

For The Tacos:

- 1 medium head of romaine lettuce, chopped
- 8 flour tortillas
- 1 medium avocado, pitted, diced
- Vegan ranch as needed
- Chopped cilantro as needed

Directions:

1. Place cauliflower florets in a bowl, add garlic powder, black pepper, red chili powder, olive oil, and ¼ cup buffalo sauce and toss until combined.

2. Spread cauliflower florets on a baking sheet in a single layer and cook for 20 minutes until roasted, flipping halfway.

3. When done, transfer cauliflower in a large bowl, then heat remaining buffalo sauce, add to cauliflower florets and toss until combined.

4. Assemble tacos and for this, top tortilla with cauliflower, lettuce, and avocado, drizzle with ranch dressing and then top with green onions.

5. Serve straight away.

Pumpkin Penne

Preparation time: 10 minutes

Cooking time: 60 minutes

Servings: 4

Ingredients:

- ½ of medium white onion, sliced into wedges
- 2 cloves of garlic, unpeeled
- 1 cup cooked and mashed sugar pie pumpkin
- ½ cup unsalted cashews, soaked, drained
- ½ teaspoon of sea salt
- 1/3 teaspoon ground black pepper
- 5 fresh sage leaves
- 2 tablespoons olive oil and more as needed for drizzling
- 1 cup vegetable broth
- 16 ounces penne pasta, cooked

Directions:

1. Take a baking sheet, place onion, pumpkin and garlic in it, drizzle with salt, season with salt and black pepper, pierce

pumpkin with a fork, cover the baking sheet and bake for 45 minutes until vegetables are very tender.

2. Then add sage in the last five minutes and after 45 minutes of baking, uncover the baking sheet and continue baking for 15 minutes.

3. When done, peel the pumpkin add to the food processor along with remaining vegetables and ingredients, except for pasta and puree until blended.

4. Place pasta in a pot, add half of the blended pumpkin mixture, stir until coated, then stir in remaining pumpkin mixture and serve.

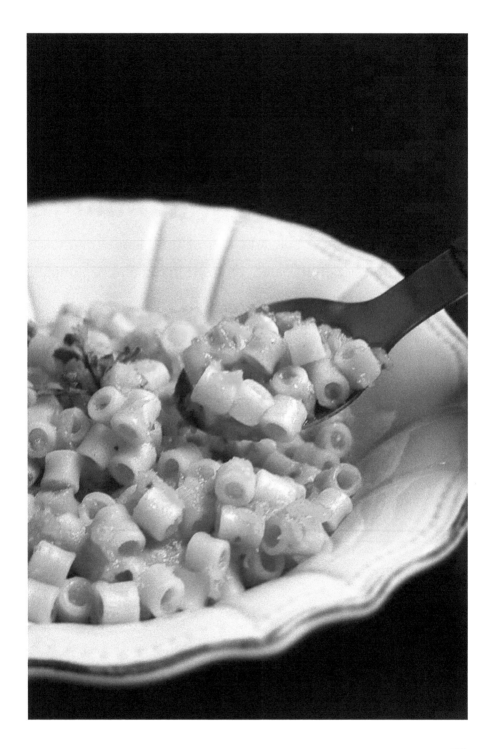

Sweet Potato Fries

Preparation time: 10 minutes

Cooking time: 30 minutes

Servings: 4

Ingredients:

- 3 large sweet potatoes
- 1/2 teaspoon sea salt
- ¼ teaspoon cayenne pepper
- 1 teaspoon cumin
- 1/4 teaspoon paprika
- 1 tablespoon olive oil

Directions:

1. Peel the potatoes, cut into wedges lengthwise, place them in a bowl, drizzle with oil and toss until combined.
2. Stir together remaining ingredients, sprinkle over sweet potatoes, spread the potatoes evenly on a baking sheet greased with oil in a single layer, and bake for 30 minutes at 400 degrees F until done, tossing twice.
3. Serve straight away.

Roasted Cauliflower

Preparation time: 10 minutes

Cooking time: 1 hour and 20 minutes

Servings: 4

Ingredients:

- 1 medium head of cauliflower
- ½ teaspoon salt
- 1 teaspoon dried parsley
- 1 teaspoon dried dill
- 1 teaspoon dried mint
- 1 tablespoon zaatar spice
- 2 tablespoons olive oil, divided
- 1 cup of water

Directions:

1. Trim the cauliflower, then slice from the bottom, drizzle it with 1 tablespoon oil, season with salt and zaatar spice, cover cauliflower with a foil and bake for 55 minutes.

2. When done, uncover the cauliflower, drizzle with remaining oil and bake for 30 minutes until roasted, turning halfway.
3. When done, sprinkle with parsley, dill, and milk and serve cauliflower with lemon wedges and tahini sauce.

Quinoa Cakes

Preparation time: 20 minutes

Cooking time: 25 minutes

Servings: 4

Ingredients:

For the Quinoa Cakes:

- 1 cup quinoa, rinsed
- 1 teaspoon garlic powder
- 1/2 teaspoon salt
- 1 teaspoon cumin
- 1/2 teaspoon Italian dried herbs
- 1 lemon, zested
- 2 teaspoons olive oil
- 2 cups of water
- 1/4 cup chopped parsley

For the Tomato Chickpea Relish:

- 1 ½ cup cooked chickpeas
- 1/4 cup chopped scallions
- 2 cups grape tomatoes, halved

- 1/4 cup chopped fresh basil
- 1 cup cucumber, diced
- ¼ teaspoon minced garlic
- 1/4 teaspoon salt
- 3 tablespoons balsamic vinegar
- 3 tablespoons olive oil

Directions:

1. Take a pot over high heat, add all the ingredients for quinoa in it except for lime zest and parsley, stir, bring the mixture to boil, then switch heat to the low level and simmer for 20 minutes.
2. Meanwhile, prepare tomato relish and for this, place all its ingredients in a bowl and stir until combined.
3. When quinoa has cooked, let it stand for 5 minutes, then fluff it with a fork, cool it for 15 minutes, stir in parsley and lemon zest and shape the mixture into four balls.
4. Fry the balls over medium heat on a greased pan for 5 minutes until browned, then transfer them on a plate, top with chickpea relish and serve.

Vibrant Salad

Preparation time: 5 minutes

Cooking time: 15 minutes

Servings: 4

Ingredients:

- 2 medium zucchini, sliced into ½-inch sliced moons
- 1 large eggplant, cut into ½-inch pieces
- 2 medium tomatoes, cut into ¾-inch wedges
- 1 red bell pepper, sliced into ½-inch strips
- 1 medium white onion, sliced
- 12 cloves of garlic, peeled
- 1 teaspoon salt
- 1 teaspoon balsamic vinegar
- 1/3 teaspoon ground black pepper
- 3 tablespoons rosemary and thyme
- Olive oil as needed

Directions:

1. Prepare all the vegetables, then spread them in a single layer on a greased sheet pan, add garlic and herbs, drizzle with oil, toss until coated and season with salt with black pepper.
2. Toss the vegetables, roast them for 40 minutes at 400 degrees F, tossing halfway, and then continue roasting for 20 minutes at 300 degrees F until tender.
3. When done, taste to adjust salt, drizzle with vinegar and serve.

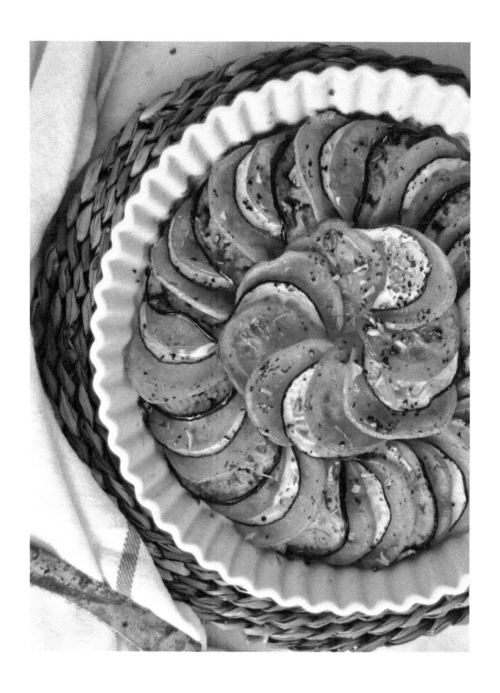

Blackened Tempeh

Preparation time: 10 minutes

Cooking time: 10 minutes

Servings: 2

Ingredients:

For the Ranch Dressing:

- 1 teaspoon Cajun spice blend
- 1/3 cup vegan ranch dressing

For the Blackened Tempeh:

- 4 radishes, sliced
- 3 cups shredded kale
- 1 medium avocado, pitted, sliced
- 1 block of tempeh
- 3 tablespoons Cajun Spice
- ½ a lemon, zested
- ¼ cup pickled onions
- ¼ teaspoon salt
- 1 teaspoon peanut oil
- 2 tablespoons olive oil

- 1 scallion, sliced

Directions:

1. Prepare the ranch dressing and for this, place all its ingredients in a bowl and stir until combined, set aside until required.
2. Take a sauté pan, place it over medium heat, add tempeh, pour in salted water to cover it, and simmer for 8 minutes until its bitterness has reduced.
3. When done, transfer tempeh to a cutting board, then cut it ½-inch slices and season with Cajun spices until coated on both sides.
4. Place shredded kale in a bowl, drizzle with peanut oil, season with salt and lemon zest, massage with fingers, then add remaining ingredients along with ranch dressing and toss until coated.
5. Distribute the kale salad between the bowl, top with tempeh and scallions and then serve.

Szechuan Tofu and Veggies

Preparation time: 10 minutes

Cooking time: 20 minutes

Servings: 2

Ingredients:

- 8 ounces tofu, drained, cubed
- 1 cup shredded carrots
- 4 ounces sliced mushrooms
- ½ cup sliced white onion
- 2 cups shredded cabbage
- 1 cup asparagus
- ½ of medium red bell pepper, cored, sliced
- 8 dried red Chinese chilies, small
- 1/3 teaspoon ground black pepper
- 2/3 teaspoon salt
- 2 tablespoons olive oil

For Garnish:

- Chopped scallions as needed
- Sesame seeds as needed
- Red chili flakes as needed

- ¼ cup Szechuan Sauce Zucchini noodles as needed for serving

Directions:

1. Take a large skillet pan, place it over medium heat, add oil, season with salt and black pepper, then season tofu with ½ teaspoon, add it to the pan in an even layer and cook for 5 minutes until golden on both sides.
2. Transfer tofu pieces to a plate, switch heat to medium-high level, add onion and mushrooms, cook for 3 minutes, then switch heat to medium level, add remaining vegetables along with chilies, toss until mixed and cook for 5 minutes until tender-crisp.
3. Pour in the sauce, toss until coated, cook for 2 minutes, then add tofu pieces, stir until coated, and cook for 2 minutes until warm.
4. When done, sprinkle with scallions and sesame seeds and serve over zucchini noodles.

Lentil Meatballs with Coconut Curry Sauce

Preparation time: 15 minutes

Cooking time: 60 minutes

Servings: 14

Ingredients:

For the Lentil Meatballs:

- 6 ounces tofu, firm, drained
- 1 cup black lentils
- ½ cup quinoa
- 1 teaspoon garlic powder
- 1 teaspoon salt
- 1/3 cup chopped cilantro
- 1 teaspoon fennel seed
- 1 Tablespoon olive oil

For the Curry:

- 1 large tomato, diced
- 2 teaspoons minced garlic
- 1 tablespoon grated ginger

- 1 teaspoon brown sugar
- ½ teaspoon ground turmeric
- ¼ teaspoon cayenne pepper
- ½ teaspoon salt
- ¼ teaspoon ground black pepper
- 1 tablespoon lime juice
- 2 tablespoons olive oil
- 1 tablespoon dried fenugreek leaves
- 13.5 ounces coconut milk, unsweetened

Directions:

1. Boil lentils and fennel in 3 cups water over high heat, then simmer for 25 minutes, and when done, drain them and set aside until required.
2. Meanwhile, boil the quinoa in 1 cup water over high heat and then simmer for 15 minutes over low heat until cooked.
3. Prepare the sauce and for this, place a pot over medium heat, add oil, ginger, and garlic, cook for 2 minutes, then stir in turmeric, cook for 1 minute, add tomatoes and cook for 5 minutes.
4. Add remaining ingredients for the sauce, stir until mixed and simmer until ready to serve.
5. Transfer half of the lentils in a food processor, add quinoa and pulse until the mixture resembles sand.

6. Tip the mixture into a bowl, add remaining ingredients for the meatballs and stir until well mixed.

7. Place tofu in a food processor, add 1 tablespoon oil, process until the smooth paste comes together, add to lentil mixture, stir until well mixed and shape the mixture into small balls.

8. Place the balls on a baking sheet, spray with oil and bake for 20 minutes until golden brown.

9. Add balls into the warm sauce, toss until coated, sprinkle with cilantro, and serve.

Stir-Fry Tofu with Mushrooms and Broccoli

Preparation time: 5 minutes

Cooking time: 12 minutes

Servings: 2

Ingredients:

- 10 ounces tofu, pressed, drained, cubed
- 8 ounces broccoli florets, steamed
- 8 ounces shiitake mushrooms, destemmed, sliced
- 1 medium shallot, peeled, diced
- 5 dried red chilies
- 2 ½ teaspoons minced garlic
- 2/3 teaspoon salt
- 2 tablespoons black vinegar, sweetened
- 2 tablespoons chopped peanuts
- 2 tablespoons soy sauce
- 2 tablespoons peanut oil
- 2 tablespoons water

For the Garnish:

- Sliced scallions as needed
- Sesame seeds as needed

Directions:

1. Take a skillet pan, place it over medium-high heat, add oil and when hot, add some and black pepper, then add tofu cubes and cook for 6 minutes until browned on all sides.
2. When done, transfer tofu cubes to a plate, add garlic and shallots, cook for 2 minutes, then add mushrooms and cook for 3 minutes until tender, add nuts and chilies, and cook for 1 minute.
3. Stir in soy sauce, vinegar and water, add steamed broccoli, toss until well coated, add tofu, toss until mixed, season with salt, and garnish with scallion and sesame seeds.
4. Serve straight away

Roasted Spaghetti Squash with Mushrooms

Preparation time: 10 minutes

Cooking time: 60 minutes

Servings: 4

Ingredients:

- 2 pounds spaghetti squash, halved
- 1 tablespoon unsalted butter
- 2 tablespoons olive oil
- ½ of a white onion, peeled, chopped
- 16 ounces sliced cremini mushrooms
- 2 teaspoons minced garlic
- 3 tablespoons sage
- 2/3 teaspoon salt
- 1/3 teaspoon ground black pepper
- 1/8 teaspoon nutmeg
- ¼ cup grated vegan parmesan cheese

Directions:

1. Bake squash on a parchment-lined baking sheet or 50 minutes at 400 degrees F until tender.
2. Meanwhile, take a large skillet pan, place it medium-high heat, add oil and butter and when hot, add onion and cook for 3 minutes until tender.
3. Then add mushrooms, switch heat to medium level, and cook for 7 minutes.
4. Stir in sage and garlic, cook for 4 minutes until mushrooms have turned brown, and then season with black pepper, nutmeg and salt.
5. When squash has roasted, pierce it with a fork, let it cool for 10 minutes, then remove its seeds and scoop the flesh of the squash to a saucepan.
6. Add mushrooms, stir until mixed, season with some more salt, and stir in cheese until incorporated.
7. Serve straight away.

Avocado Linguine

Preparation time: 10 minutes

Cooking time: 0 minute

Servings: 4

Ingredients:

- ½ cup arugula
- 2 medium avocados
- 2 cloves of garlic, peeled
- 1/4 teaspoon ground white pepper
- 3/4 teaspoons salt
- 1 teaspoon lemon zest
- 3 tablespoons lemon juice
- 3 tablespoons olive oil
- 8 ounces linguine, whole-wheat, boiled

Directions:

1. Prepare the avocado sauce, and for this, place all the ingredients in a food processor, except for pasta, arugula, pepper, and lemon zest and pulse until smooth.

2. Tip the puree in a large bowl, add remaining ingredients, toss until well mixed and taste to adjust seasoning.

3. Serve straight away.

Scallion Pancakes

Preparation time: 40 minutes

Cooking time: 8 minutes

Servings: 2

Ingredients:

- 2 large bunches of green onions, sliced
- 4 cups all-purpose flour
- 1/4 teaspoon salt
- 1/4 cup and
- 1 tablespoon olive oil
- 1 1/2 cups chilled water

Directions:

1. Place flour in a bowl, stir in water until a smooth dough comes together, knead it for 5 minutes, then cover it with plastic wrap and let it stand for 30 minutes.
2. Then roll the dough into 1/8 thick crust, brush the top with 1 tablespoon oil, season with salt, and scatter with some green onion.

3. Roll the dough into a cigar shape, roll it again into 1/8 inch thick crust and fry it into remaining hot oil for 3 minutes per side until cooked and golden.

4. When done, transfer pancake to a plate lined with paper towels, let it stand for 5 minutes, then cut it into 3 wedges and serve.

Mushroom and Broccoli Noodles

Preparation time: 10 minutes

Cooking time: 10 minutes

Servings: 4

Ingredients:

- 2 linguine pasta, whole-grain, cooked
- 8 ounces chestnut mushroom, sliced
- 4 spring onions, sliced
- 1 small head of broccoli, cut into florets, steamed
- ½ teaspoon minced garlic
- ½ teaspoon red chili flakes
- 1 tablespoon sesame oil
- 2 teaspoons hoisin sauce
- ¼ cup roasted cashew
- 3 tablespoons stock

Directions:

1. Take a large frying pan, place it over medium heat, add oil and when hot, add mushrooms and cook for 2 minutes until golden.

2. Stir in garlic, onion and chili flakes, cook for 1 minute, stir in broccoli and toss in pasta until hot.
3. Drizzle with hoisin sauce and 3 tablespoons of stock, toss until mixed, cook for 1 minute and remove the pan from heat.
4. Top with cashews, drizzle with some more sesame oil and serve.

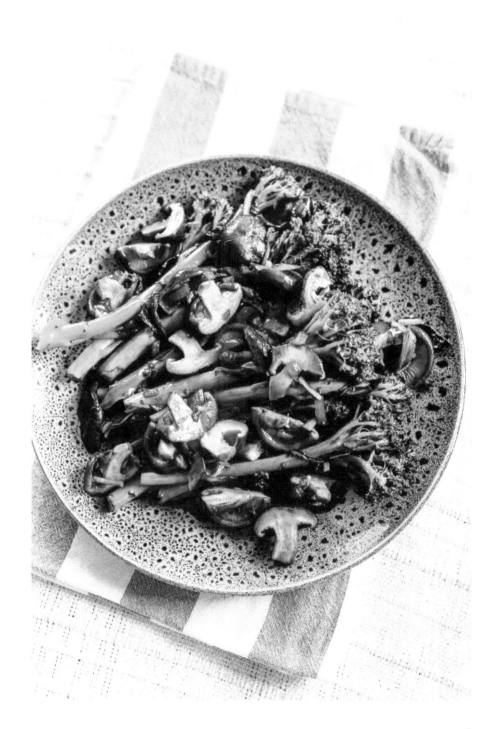

Pasta with Creamy Greens and Lemon

Preparation time: 5 minutes

Cooking time: 10 minutes

Servings: 4

Ingredients:

- 5 ounces broccoli, cut into florets
- 3.5 ounces frozen soya beans
- ¼ cup basil leaves
- 3.5 ounces frozen peas
- 3.5 ounces mange tout
- 2/3 teaspoon salt
- 1/3 teaspoon ground black pepper
- 1 lemon, juiced, zested
- 5.3 ounces vegan mascarpone
- 3 ounces grated vegan parmesan cheese
- 12 ounces whole-grain pasta, cooked

Directions:

1. Cook the pasta in a saucepan, add all the vegetables in the last 3 minutes, and, when done, drain the pasta and vegetables.
2. Return the pasta and vegetables into the pan, add remaining ingredients and stir until well combined.
3. Serve straight away

Dijon Maple Burgers

Serves: 12

Time: 50 Minutes

Ingredients:

- 1 Red Bell Pepper
- 19 Ounces Can Chickpeas, Rinsed & Drained
- 1 Cup Almonds, Ground
- 2 Teaspoons Dijon Mustard
- 1 Teaspoon Oregano
- ½ Teaspoon Sage
- 1 Cup Spinach, Fresh
- 1 – ½ Cups Rolled Oats
- 1 Clove Garlic, Pressed
- ½ Lemon, Juiced
- 2 Teaspoons Maple Syrup, Pure

Directions:

1. Get out a baking sheet.
2. Line it with parchment paper.
3. Cut your red pepper in half and then take the seeds out.

4. Place it on your baking sheet, and roast in the oven while you prepare your other ingredients.
5. Process your chickpeas, almonds, mustard and maple syrup together in a food processor.
6. Add in your lemon juice, oregano, sage, garlic and spinach, processing again.
7. Make sure it's combined, but don't puree it.
8. Once your red bell pepper is softened, which should roughly take ten minutes, add this to the processor as well.
9. Add in your oats, mixing well.
10. Form twelve patties, cooking in the oven for a half hour.
11. They should be browned.

Flavorful Refried Beans

Servings: 8

Preparation time: 8 hours and 15 minutes

Ingredients:

- 3 cups of pinto beans, rinsed
- 1 small jalapeno pepper, seeded and chopped
- 1 medium-sized white onion, peeled and sliced
- 2 tablespoons of minced garlic
- 5 teaspoons of salt
- 2 teaspoons of ground black pepper
- 1/4 teaspoon of ground cumin
- 9 cups of water

Directions:

1. Using a 6-quarts slow cooker, place all the ingredients and stir until it mixes properly.
2. Cover the top, plug in the slow cooker; adjust the cooking time to 6 hours, let it cook on high heat setting and add more water if the beans get too dry.

3. When the beans are done, drain them and reserve the liquid.
4. Mash the beans using a potato masher and pour in the reserved cooking liquid until it reaches your desired mixture.
5. Serve immediately.

Spicy Black-Eyed Peas

Servings: 8

Preparation time: 8 hours and 20 minutes

Ingredients:

- 32-ounce black-eyed peas, uncooked
- 1 cup of chopped orange bell pepper
- 1 cup of chopped celery
- 8-ounce of chipotle peppers, chopped
- 1 cup of chopped carrot
- 1 cup of chopped white onion
- 1 teaspoon of minced garlic
- 3/4 teaspoon of salt
- 1/2 teaspoon of ground black pepper
- 2 teaspoons of liquid smoke flavoring
- 2 teaspoons of ground cumin
- 1 tablespoon of adobo sauce
- 2 tablespoons of olive oil
- 1 tablespoon of apple cider vinegar
- 4 cups of vegetable broth

Directions:

1. Place a medium-sized non-stick skillet pan over an average temperature of heat; add the bell peppers, carrot, onion, garlic, oil and vinegar.
2. Stir until it mixes properly and let it cook for 5 to 8 minutes or until it gets translucent.
3. Transfer this mixture to a 6-quarts slow cooker and add the peas, chipotle pepper, adobo sauce and the vegetable broth.
4. Stir until mixes properly and cover the top.
5. Plug in the slow cooker; adjust the cooking time to 8 hours and let it cook on the low heat setting or until peas are soft.
6. Serve right away.

Tomato Artichoke Soup

Preparation time: 5 minutes

Cooking time: 35 minutes

Servings: 4

Ingredients:

- 1 can artichoke hearts, drained
- 1 can diced tomatoes, undrained
- 3 cups vegetable broth
- 1 small onion, chopped
- 2 cloves garlic, crushed
- 1 tbsp pesto black pepper, to taste

Directions:

1. Combine all ingredients in the slow cooker.
2. Cover and cook on low for 8-10 hours or on high for 4-5 hours.
3. Blend the soup in batches and return it to the slow cooker.
4. Season with salt and pepper to taste and serve.

Mushroom Salad

Preparation time: 10 minutes

Cooking time: 20 minutes

Servings: 2

Ingredients:

- 1 tbsp. butter
- ½ pound cremini mushrooms, chopped
- 2 tbsp. extra virgin olive oil
- Salt and black pepper to taste
- 2 bunches arugula
- 4 slices prosciutto
- 1 tbsp. apple cider vinegar
- 4 sundried tomatoes in oil, drained and chopped
- Parmesan cheese, shaved
- Fresh parsley leaves, chopped

Directions:

1. Heat a pan with butter and half of the oil.
2. Add the mushrooms, salt, and pepper.
3. Stir-fry for 3 minutes.

4. Reduce heat.
5. Stir again, and cook for 3 minutes more.
6. Add rest of the oil and vinegar.
7. Stir and cook for 1 minute.
8. Place arugula on a platter, add prosciutto on top, add the mushroom mixture, sundried tomatoes, more salt and pepper, parmesan shavings, parsley, and serve.

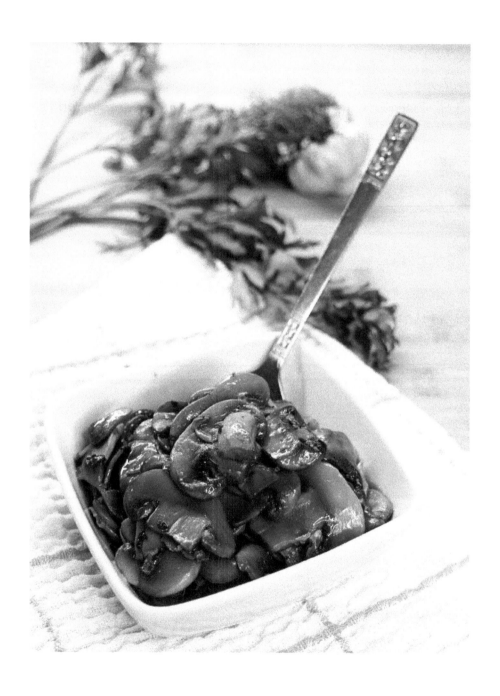

October Potato Soup

Preparation time: 5 minutes

Cooking time: 20 minutes 3 servings.

Ingredients:

- 4 minced garlic cloves
- 2 tsp. coconut oil
- 3 diced celery stalks
- 1 diced onion
- 2 tsp. yellow mustard seeds
- 5 diced Yukon potatoes
- 6 cups vegetable broth
- 1 tsp. oregano
- 1 tsp. paprika
- ½ tsp. cayenne pepper
- 1 tsp. chili powder
- salt and pepper to taste

Directions:

1. Begin by sautéing the garlic and the mustard seeds together in the oil in a large soup pot.

2. Next, add the onion and sauté the mixture for another five minutes.

3. Add the celery, the broth, the potatoes, and all the spices, and continue to stir.

4. Allow the soup to simmer for thirty minutes without a cover.

5. Next, Position about three cups of the soup in a blender, and puree the soup until you've reached a smooth consistency.

6. Pour this back into the big soup pot, stir, and serve warm.

7. Enjoy.

Lentil Luxury Soup

Preparation time: 5 minutes

Cooking time: 50 minutes

4 Servings.

Ingredients:

- 5 minced garlic cloves
- 1 tsp. olive oil
- 1 diced onion
- ½ tsp. coriander
- 1 cup diced celery
- 1 tsp. cumin
- ½ tsp. cayenne pepper
- 6 cups vegetable broth
- ¾ cup red lentils
- ¼ cup black lentils
- 1 ¼ cup green lentils
- salt and pepper to taste

Directions:

1. Begin by heating the oil, the garlic, and the onion in the bottom of the soup pot for eight minutes.
2. Next, add the celery and the spices.
3. Cook for three more minutes.
4. Add the cooked or canned lentils to the soup pot, next. Pour in the broth and stir well.
5. Next, allow the soup to simmer for forty-five minutes.
6. Stir often.
7. Salt and pepper the soup as you please, and serve warm.
8. Enjoy.

Exotic Butternut Squash and Chickpea Curry

Servings: 8

Preparation time: 6 hours and 15 minutes

Ingredients:

- 1 1/2 cups of shelled peas
- 1 1/2 cups of chick peas, uncooked and rinsed
- 2 1/2 cups of diced butternut squash
- 12 ounce of chopped spinach
- 2 large tomatoes, diced
- 1 small white onion, peeled and chopped
- 1 teaspoon of minced garlic
- 1 teaspoon of salt
- 3 tablespoons of curry powder
- 14-ounce of coconut milk
- 3 cups of vegetable broth
- 1/4 cup of chopped cilantro

Directions:

- Using a 6-quarts slow cooker, place all the ingredients into it except for the spinach and peas.
- Cover the top, plug in the slow cooker; adjust the cooking time to 6 hours and let it cook on the high heat setting or until the chickpeas get tender.
- 30 minutes to ending your cooking, add the peas and spinach to the slow cooker and let it cook for the remaining 30 minutes.
- Stir to check the sauce, if the sauce is runny, stir in a mixture of a tablespoon of cornstarch mixed with 2 tablespoons of water.
- Serve with boiled rice.

Collard Greens And Tomatoes

Preparation Time: 10 minutes

Cooking Time: 10 minutes

Servings: 9

Ingredients

- 1 pound collard greens
- ¼ cup cherry tomatoes, halved
- 1 tablespoon apple cider vinegar
- 2 tablespoons veggie stock
- Salt and black pepper to the taste

Directions:

1. In a pan that fits your Air Fryer, combine tomatoes, collard greens, vinegar, stock, salt and pepper, stir, introduce in your Air Fryer and cook at 320 ° F for 10 minutes.
2. Divide between plates and serve as a side dish.

Creamy Artichoke and Horseradish Soup

Preparation time: 5 minutes

Cooking time: 50 minutes

Servings: 4

Ingredients:

- 1 can artichoke hearts, drained
- 3 cups vegetable broth
- 1 tbsp vegan horseradish sauce
- 2 tbsp lemon juice
- 1 small onion, finely cut
- 2 cloves garlic, crushed
- 3 tbsp olive oil
- 2 tbsp flour
- 2 tbsp chopped fresh chives plus extra to garnish

Directions:

1. Gently sauté the onion and garlic in some olive oil.

2. Add in the flour, whisking constantly, and then add the hot vegetable broth slowly, while still whisking.
3. Cook for about 5 minutes.
4. Blend the artichokes, salt and pepper until smooth.
5. Add the puree to the broth mix, stir well, and then stir in the horseradish sauce and chopped chives.
6. Ladle the soup into bowls and serve.

Celery Root Soup

Preparation time: 5 minutes

Cooking time: 20 minutes

Servings: 4

Ingredients:

- 2 leeks (white and light green parts only), chopped
- 2 garlic cloves, crushed
- 1 large celery root, peeled and diced
- 2 potatoes, peeled and diced
- 4 cups vegetable broth
- 1 bay leaf
- 2 tbsp olive oil salt and black pepper, to taste

Directions:

1. In a skillet, heat olive oil, then add the leeks and sauté about 3-4 minutes.
2. Add in the garlic and sauté an additional 3-40 seconds.
3. In a slow cooker, add the sautéed leeks and garlic, celeriac, potatoes, broth, bay leaf, salt, and pepper.
4. Cover and cook on low heat for 7-8 hours.

5. Set aside to cool, remove the bay leaf, then process in a blender or with an immersion blender until smooth.

Quizzical Quinoa Soup

Preparation time: 5 minutes

Cooking time: 20 minutes

6 Servings.

Ingredients:

- 1 diced onion
- 1 tbsp. olive oil
- 6 diced carrots
- 3 minced garlic cloves
- 1 cup quinoa
- 16 ounces pink beans
- 32 ounces vegetable broth
- 2 tsp. curry powder
- 1 tsp. paprika
- 2 tsp. curry powder
- 1/3 cup chopped dill
- 5 ounces spinach leaves
- salt and pepper to taste

Directions:

1. Begin by heating the oil and the vegetables together in the bottom of a soup pot for about seven minutes.
2. Next, add the vegetable broth, the quinoa, the beans, and all the spices.
3. Simmer this mixture for twenty minutes with the cover on.
4. Next, add the tomatoes and a bit more water to administer the proper soup texture.
5. Cook the mixture for ten more minutes.
6. Next, add the parsley, stir for a few minutes, and then serve the soup instantly.
7. Enjoy!

Barley Country Living Soup

Preparation time: 5 minutes

Cooking time: 30 minutes

8 Servings.

Ingredients:

- 2 tbsp. olive oil
- 32 ounces vegetable broth
- 1 diced onion
- 2 diced celery stalks
- 4 diced carrots
- 1 ¼ cup pearl barley
- 12 ounces sliced mushrooms
- 1 tbsp. basil
- 2 cups soymilk
- 1/3 cup minced parsley
- salt and pepper to taste

Directions:

1. Bring by heating the oil and the vegetables together in a soup pot for eight minutes.
2. Next, add the broth, the barley, and the spices to the mixture.
3. Allow the mixture to simmer for fifty minutes with a cover on top.
4. Make sure to stir occasionally.
5. Next, add the soymilk, and season the soup with salt and pepper.
6. Make sure to allow the soup to rest for thirty minutes prior to serving in order to allow it to thicken.
7. Enjoy.

Mediterranean Garbanzo-Bean Fritters

Preparation time: 10 minutes

Cooking time: 25 minutes

Servings: 4.

Ingredients:

- 1 cup garbanzo bean flour
- 1 tsp. salt
- ½ tsp. cumin
- 1 ¼ cup chopped spinach
- ¼ tsp. baking soda
- 4 minced garlic cloves
- 2 sliced scallions
- 1 cup drained garbanzo beans
- 1 cup olive oil

Directions:

1. Begin by preheating the oven to 200 degrees Fahrenheit.
2. Next, stir together the flour, salt, and cumin.

3. Add hot water a little bit at a time in order to create a paste-like texture: like pancake batter.
4. Allow this mixture to stand at room temperature for one hour.
5. Afterwards, add the baking soda, the garlic, and the spinach to the mixture.
6. Stir.
7. Next, add the scallions and the chickpeas.
8. Pour the olive oil in the skillet, and place the heat on medium.
9. When you've heated the oil sufficiently, place the fritters on the oil and brown them for three minutes on each side.
10. Drain the fritters on paper towels, and serve them with your favorite dipping sauce.

Asian-Inspired Summer Goi Cuan

Preparation time: 10 minutes

Cooking time: 30 minutes

24 rolls.

Ingredients:

- 24 round rice paper wrappers
- 6-7 cups of jasmine tea
- 2 de-ribbed and separated lettuce heads
- 9 ounces cooked thin rice vermicelli noodles
- ½ cup Thai basil leaves
- 1 ½ cups enoki mushrooms
- 1 cup chopped mint
- ¼ cup chopped cilantro
- ½ cup sliced scallions
- 2 sliced carrots
- 1 sliced cucumber

Directions:

1. Begin by preparing the tea and keeping it warm.
2. Next, dip each of the rice paper wrappers into the tea.
3. Place the rice wrappers on a cutting board, and place a layer of lettuce in the center.
4. Enter in a bit of all of the above ingredients.
5. Next, fold over the bottom of the rice paper overtop of the filling.
6. Tuck in the sides, and continue to wrap the rice up.
7. Do this for each of the 24 rice paper wrappers, and chill the rolls prior to serving.
8. Enjoy!

Yummy Roasted Mushrooms

Preparation time: 10 minutes

Cooking time: 30 minutes

8 Servings.

Ingredients:

- 2 pounds cremini mushrooms
- 2 ½ tbsp. olive oil
- 2 tbsp. soy sauce
- 2 minced garlic cloves
- spinach for serving

Directions:

1. Begin by preheating the oven to 350 degrees Fahrenheit.
2. Slice up the mushrooms, and place the mushrooms in a large mixing bowl with the rest of the ingredients—except for the spinach.
3. Bake the ingredients in a baking dish for thirty minutes. Next, remove the baked ingredients, and place them overtop of the spinach in a serving bowl.
4. Enjoy.

Savory Scallion Pancakes

Preparation time: 10 minutes

Cooking time: 20 minutes

24 mini pancakes.

Ingredients:

- 1 cup spelt flour
- 1 cup and
- 2 tbsp. rice milk
- 1 cup sliced scallions
- 1 tsp. salt
- olive oil for cooking

Directions:

1. Begin by combining the above ingredients in a mixing bowl.
2. Stir the ingredients well until they're smooth.
3. Afterwards, oil up a griddle and place about 1/8 of a cup of batter on the griddle for each pancake.
4. Cook each side of the pancake to achieve a golden brown color.

5. Next, place the pancakes on a plate, and cover the pancakes while you continue to cook the rest of the batter.
6. Place the pancakes out on a nice platter, and serve warm.

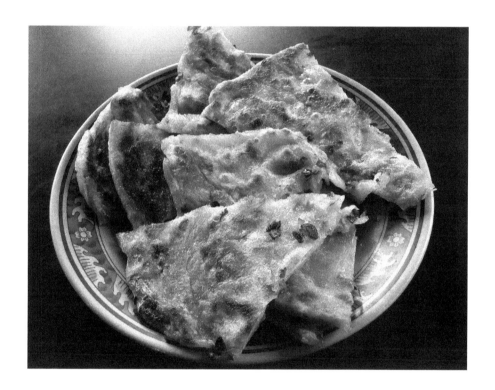

Smokin' Peanut and Tofu

Preparation time: 10 minutes

Cooking time: 60 minutes 10 servings.

Ingredients:

- 7 ounces smoked tofu
- 6 celery stalks
- 2 ounces roasted peanuts
- 3 tbsp. chili oil
- ½ tsp. sugar salt to taste

Directions:

1. Begin by slicing the tofu into small cubes and squeezing them of their water.
2. Afterwards, slice up the celery into small strips the same size as the small tofu squares.
3. Allow water to boil in a small saucepan.
4. Add the celery and allow it to blanch for one minute.
5. Afterwards, remove the celery and allow it to cool. Shake it dry.

6. Bring all the above ingredients together in a bowl for an essential appetizer.

7. Enjoy!

Artichoke Attack Appetizer

Preparation time: 10 minutes

Cooking time: 40 minutes

6 Servings.

Ingredients:

- 10 ounces asparagus
- 8 ounces button mushrooms
- 8 ounces artichoke hearts
- 1 chopped dill pickle
- 1 sliced zucchini
- ¼ cup chopped parsley
- ½ cup vegan mayonnaise (recipe here)
- 1 juiced lemon
- salt and pepper to taste

Directions:

1. Begin by slicing up the mushrooms and placing them in a skillet with about ¼cup water.
2. Cover the skillet and allow them to steam on medium-heat for two and a half minutes.

3. Next, drain the mushrooms and allow them to cool.
4. To the side, trim at the bottom of the asparagus, and slice the asparagus into smaller, one-inch pieces.
5. Place the asparagus in the mushroom skillet, and place just about three tbsp. of water at the bottom.
6. Steam the asparagus until the asparagus is a bright green.
7. Drain the asparagus, and rinse it.
8. Bring the mushrooms and asparagus together in a serving bowl.
9. Bring in the artichoke hearts, the dill pickle, the zucchini, the parsley, the mayonnaise, the lemon, and the salt and pepper.
10. Mix well, and enjoy.

Lucky Lemon Mushrooms

Preparation time: 10 minutes

Cooking time: 20 minutes

6 Servings.

Ingredients:

- 1 tsp. agave nectar
- 3 tbsp. lemon juice
- 1 tbsp. olive oil
- 2 minced garlic cloves
- 10 ounces sliced portabella mushrooms

Directions:

1. Bring together the agave nectar, the lemon juice, the olive oil, and the minced garlic in a mixing bowl.
2. Place the sliced mushrooms in the created mixture, and stir them together. Next, place the mushrooms in a baking pan, and pour the marinade overtop of them.
3. Broil the mushrooms for four minutes.
4. After four minutes, stir the mushrooms.
5. Broil them for an additional five minutes.

6. The mushrooms should be darker.

7. Remove the mushrooms, and serve them warm.

8. Enjoy!

Pesto Stuffed Mushrooms

Preparation time: 20 minutes

Cooking time: 25 minutes

Servings: 6

Ingredients:

- 6 large cremini mushrooms
- 6 bacon slices
- 2 tablespoons basil pesto
- 5 tablespoons low-fat cream cheese softened

What you'll need from the store cupboard:

- None

Directions:

1. Line a cookie sheet with foil and preheat oven to 3750F.
2. In a small bowl mix well, pesto and cream cheese.
3. Remove stems of mushrooms and discard.
4. Evenly fill mushroom caps with pesto-cream cheese filling.
5. Get one stuffed mushroom and a slice of bacon.
6. Wrap the bacon all over the mushrooms.

7. Repeat process on remaining mushrooms and bacon.

8. Place bacon-wrapped mushrooms on prepared pan and bake for 25 minutes or until bacon is crispy.

9. Let it cool, evenly divide into suggested servings, and enjoy.

Delicious Potato Mix

Preparation Time: 10 minutes

Cooking Time: 25 minutes

Servings:

Ingredients

- 6 ounces jarred roasted red bell peppers, chopped
- 3 garlic cloves, minced
- 2 tablespoons parsley, chopped
- Salt and black pepper to the taste
- 2 tablespoons chives, chopped
- 4 potatoes, peeled and cut into wedges
- Cooking spray

Directions:

1. In a pan that fits your Air Fryer, combine roasted bell peppers with garlic, parsley, salt, pepper, chives, potato wedges and the oil, toss, transfer to your Air Fryer and cook at 350 °F for 25 minutes.
2. Divide between plates and serve as a side dish.

Easy Portobello Mushrooms

Preparation Time: 10 minutes

Cooking Time: 12 minutes

Servings:

Ingredients

- 4 big Portobello mushroom caps
- 1 tablespoon olive oil
- 1 cup spinach, torn
- 1/3 cup vegan breadcrumbs
- ¼ teaspoon rosemary, chopped

Directions:

1. Rub mushrooms caps with the oil, place them in your Air Fryer's basket and cook them at 350 ° F for 2 minutes.
2. Meanwhile, in a bowl, mix spinach, rosemary and breadcrumbs and stir well. Stuff mushrooms with this mix, place them in your Air Fryer's basket again and cook at 350 ° F for 10 minutes.
3. Divide them between plates and serve as a side dish.

Sweet Potatoes Side Dish

Preparation Time: 10 minutes

Cooking time: 3 hours

Servings: 10

Ingredients:

- 4 pounds sweet potatoes, thinly sliced
- 3 tablespoons stevia
- ½ cup orange juice
- ½ teaspoon sage, dried
- 2 tablespoons olive oil

Directions:

1. Arrange potato slices on the bottom of your slow cooker.
2. Add this over potatoes, cover slow cooker and cook on High for 3 hours.
3. Divide between plates and serve as a side dish.
4. Enjoy!

Wild Rice Mix

Preparation Time: 10 minutes

Cooking time: 6 hours

Servings: 12

Ingredients:

- 40 ounces veggie stock
- 2 and ½ cups wild rice
- 1 cup carrot, shredded
- 4 ounces mushrooms, sliced
- 2 tablespoons olive oil
- 2 teaspoons marjoram, dried and crushed
- Salt and black pepper to the taste
- 2/3 cup dried cherries
- ½ cup pecans, toasted and chopped
- 2/3 cup green onions, chopped

Directions:

1. In your slow cooker, mix stock with wild rice, carrot, mushrooms, oil, marjoram, salt, pepper, cherries, pecans and green onions, toss, cover and cook on Low for 6 hours.

2. Stir wild rice one more time, divide between plates and serve as a side dish.

3. Enjoy!

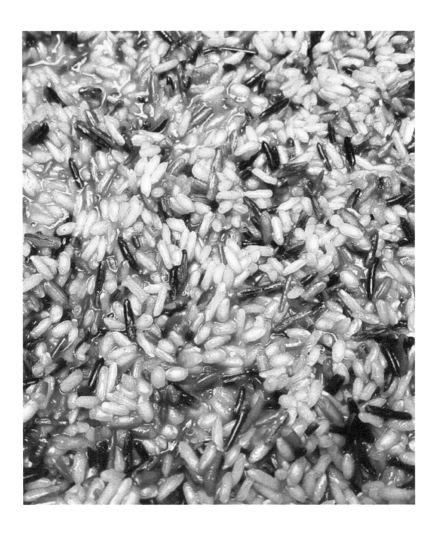

Thai Peanut Zucchini Noodle Salad

Preparation Time: 10 minutes

Cooking Time: 10 minutes

Serving Yields: 4

Ingredients:

1. Medium zucchini
2. 3 spiralized Carrot
3. 1 spiralized Chopped green onions.
4. .25 cup Extra firm tofu, drained and cubed
5. .5 of 1 block Skinny Peanut Sauce
6. 5 cup +1-2 tbsp.water
7. Peanuts 5 cup

Ingredients for the sauce:

- Protein Plus peanut flour
- .25 cup Ginger
- 1 tsp. Garlic powder
- .5 tsp. Low-sodium soy sauce gluten-free, if desired
- 2 tbsp. Lakanto Liquid Monkfruit Sweetener or another liquid sweetener

- 6 drops or to taste Lime juice
- juice of 2 limes
- 1 tbsp. Water - add more if desired
- 2 tbsp.

Ingredients for the salad:

- Spiralized carrot
- 1 Medium spiralized zucchini
- 3 Diced green onions
- .25 cup Extra-firm tofu
- .5 of a block Skinny Peanut Sauce
- .5 cup plus 1-2 Tbsp water
- Peanuts - .5 cup

Directions:

1. Drain and cube the tofu.
2. Prepare the sauce by adding the water until it's like you like it.
3. Combine the remainder of the fixings except for the peanuts in another container.
4. Top it off with the prepared salad dressing, and toss well.
5. Sprinkle using some of the peanuts, and serve.

Almond Butter Brownies

Preparation Time: 30 minutes

Serves: 4

Ingredients:

- 1 scoop protein powder
- 2 tbsp cocoa powder
- 1/2 cup almond butter, melted
- 1 cup bananas, overripe

Directions:

1. Preheat the oven to 350 F/ 176 C.
2. Spray brownie tray with cooking spray.
3. Add all Ingredients into the blender and blend until smooth.
4. Pour batter into the prepared dish and bake in preheated oven for 20 minutes.
5. Serve and enjoy.

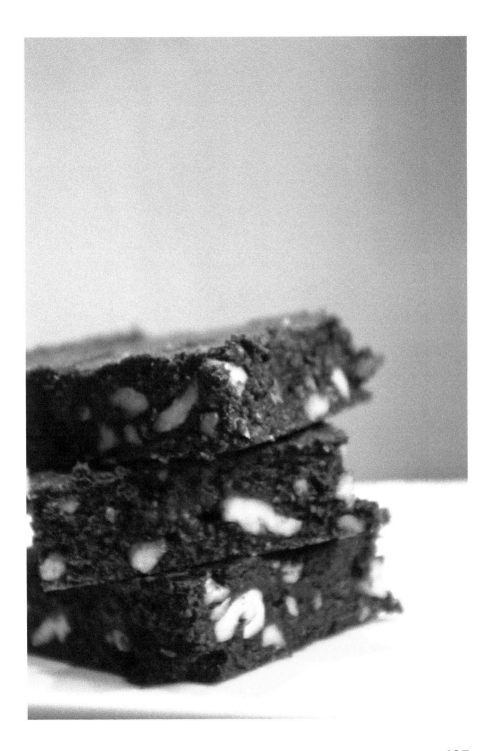